DIRECT PRIMARY CARE

THE CURE FOR OUR BROKEN HEALTHCARE SYSTEM

Paul Thomas, MD
of Plum Health DPC

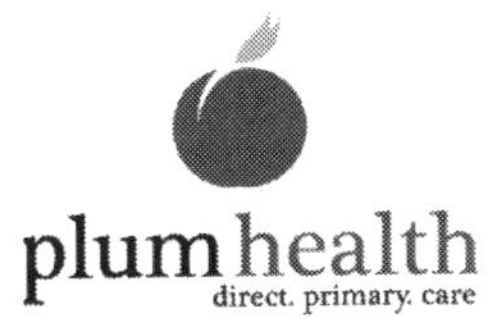

Direct Primary Care:

The Cure for Our Broken Healthcare System

by Paul Thomas, M.D.

Published in the United Sates by

Plum Health DPC, Detroit, Michigan

Paperback ISBN 978-1-7324038-0-2

Kindle ISBN 978-1-7324038-2-6

iBook ISBN 978-1-7324038-1-9

First Edition, November 2018

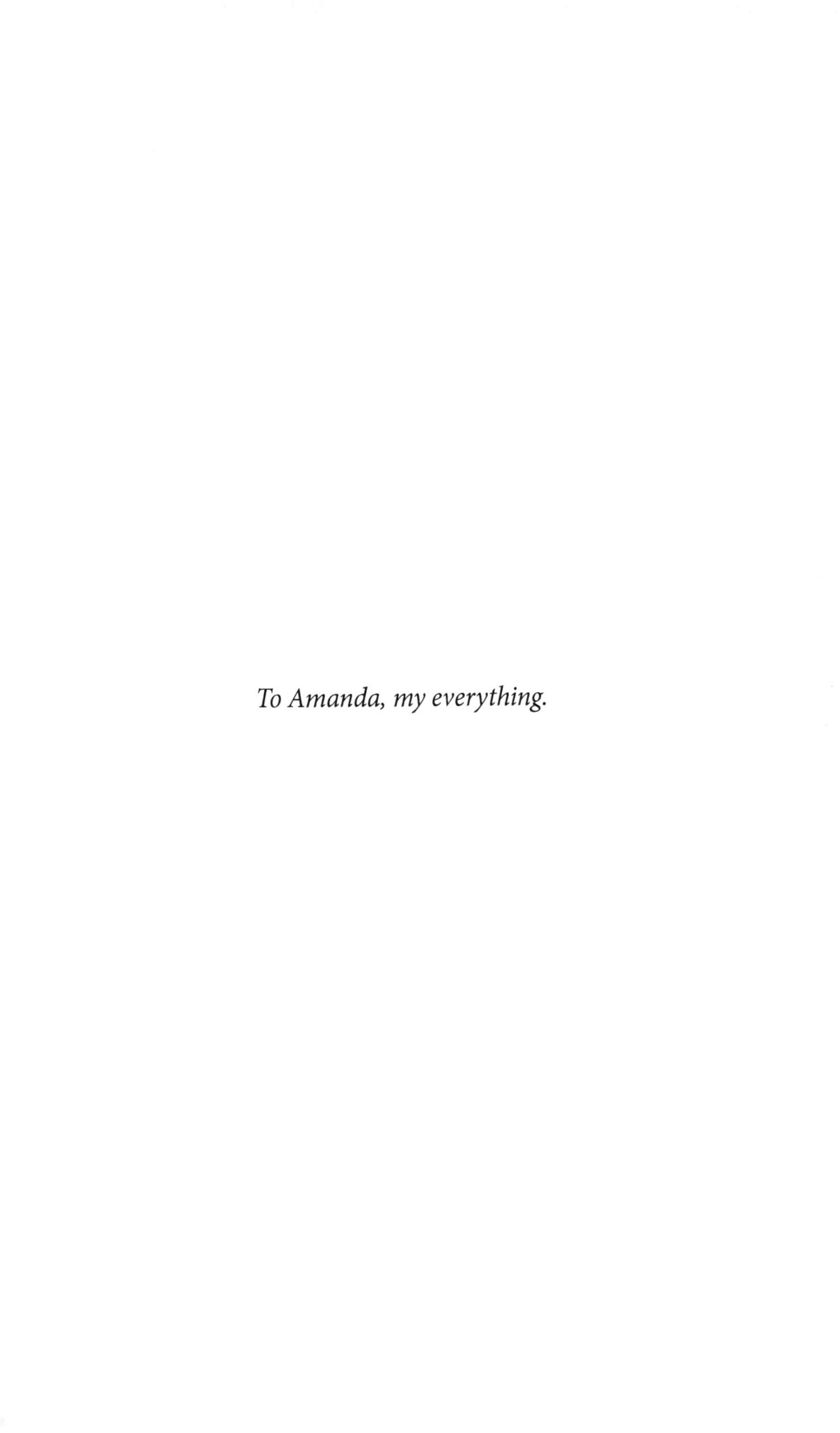

To Amanda, my everything.

"Direct Primary Care is quickly becoming an important contributor to the transformation of our nation's healthcare system and Plum Health sits at the leading edge of this revolution. A model that truly fits into the lifestyle of the patient, Plum Health's true differentiation is driven by Paul Thomas's passion and unwavering desire to promote optimal health."

Paul Riser, Director, Technology-Based Entrepreneurship @ TechTown Detroit

"Dr. Paul has eloquently described what is possible when innovative physicians break the mold and design a system that is truly patient-centric. The Direct Primary Care movement is a catalyst for reshaping the healthcare industry by creatively destroying barriers between patients and their doctors."

Dr. Josh Umbehr, CEO and Physician at AtlasMD

"Dr. Paul's sentiments resonate strongly with many of us in the healthcare profession. A thoughtful collection of solutions and a new way of practicing medicine that can offer hope for patients, and a more fulfilling career for primary care doctors."

Dr. Rami Wehbi, DO - Founder, Beyond Medicine

EPIGRAPH

"For what it's worth: it's never too late or, in my case, too early to be whoever you want to be. There's no time limit, stop whenever you want. You can change or stay the same, there are no rules to this thing. We can make the best or the worst of it. I hope you make the best of it. And I hope you see things that startle you. I hope you feel things you never felt before. I hope you meet people with a different point of view. I hope you live a life you're proud of. If you find that you're not, I hope you have the courage to start all over again."

– *F. Scott Fitzgerald*

TABLE OF CONTENTS

FOREWORD

I was sitting in my office in Leamington, Ontario, Canada, when I received an email from Nicole Mangis, founder of Brut Detroit and a well-known member of Detroit's entrepreneurial and startup community. The email was a "request to connect with" type of email, my favorite kind. This was my first introduction to Dr. Paul Thomas and Plum Health DPC.

Within a few days, Paul and I were on the phone chatting about this concept called "Direct Primary Care." As a Canadian, I had not yet heard of this type of healthcare model, and it took me a few minutes to grasp the concept because it was just so simple, I kept thinking to myself, "It has got to be more complicated than that."

Once I understood, we spent about 30 minutes discussing and brainstorming opportunities for Plum Health mainly around positioning (marketing, brand strategy, communication, public relations) and partnering to have the most significant impact in Detroit, a city that is grossly underserved when it comes to primary "everyday" health care.

To give you a little bit of background, I decided to pursue a career in health care as I recognized that I had a passion for people and service drawn out by my affinity and experience in the hospitality industry. Early on in my career, I set a mission statement for myself to "humanize the health system through innovation."I believe that we can build systems for health and wellness that are community and citizen-centric, built on evidence and not ego, and by doing so, we can build communities, where people can live long, happy, productive, meaningful and healthy lives. I believe that Plum Health DPC embodies this. It has been such a privilege to support and watch Dr. Paul Thomas sprint at bringing health to a community through service, by making health care radically accessible, radically affordable and radically human. As a health systems innovator, I am particularly fond of Dr. Thomas's use of ubiquitous digital tools (phone, email, text, Face Time) to stay compassionately connected to his patients. Plum Health is an example of how simple deployments of technology, used thoughtfully can make a world of difference to the patient experience. Currently, "hospital-based-health-insurance-company-systems" around the world are looking to re-invent themselves as their model is no longer sustainable from an economic perspective, nor is it aligned with changing consumer sentiments, demographics, and community, cultural, and political values.

As you read over the next few pages, regardless of what your role is in the healthcare industry, I hope you will be inspired like I have been to rethink how we can get back to the fundamentals of delivering human-centered care.

I am confident that Dr. Paul Thomas, Plum Health and the proponents of Direct Primary Care will play a prominent role in helping us define and shape the future of our industry.

Dr. Thomas, thank you for your leadership.

Zain Ismail
Innovator, Connector, Entrepreneur
Organizer, Hacking Health Windsor Detroit
Founding Member, Detroit Windsor MedHealth Innovation Cluster
Zainismail.com

"If I were to redesign our nation's health care system, and place patients at the center, which is where they properly belong, the foundations would be built upon the concept of Direct Primary Care and the ideals expressed in this book."

Jack D. Sobel, M.D., Dean, Wayne State University School of Medicine
and Distinguished Professor of Medicine (Infectious Disease)
and Obstetrics and Gynecology

"We spend nearly one fifth of our GDP for substandard healthcare in America. If we're going to fix it, we need to think outside the box. Direct Primary Care is part of the solution, and Dr. Paul Thomas is one of its leaders. As health director of the City of Detroit, I saw firsthand how lack of access to primary care hurt Detroiters - and I saw how Dr. Thomas's model could provide that services in an accessible, affordable, and friendly way. This book matters for anyone who believes healthcare has to change, and that revolutionizing primary care is part of that. Kudos to Dr. Thomas for his leadership in Detroit and in this movement."

Abdul El-Sayed, MD, DPhil

"Dr. Paul has perfectly encapsulated the ideals and importance of the DPC movement. If you want to understand this grassroots movement of primary care physicians and patients, read this book."

Ryan Neuhofel, DO, MPH, Family Physician, Owner of NeuCare,
President of the Direct Primary Care Alliance

PREFACE

I initially discovered Direct Primary Care while on a road trip in November 2012. I was driving back to Detroit from a residency position interview at the University of Minnesota and I listened to a podcast featuring an interview with Dr. Josh Umbehr, discussing his DPC startup in Wichita, Kansas, called Atlas MD.

It was refreshing to hear a Family Medicine doctor speaking so passionately about saving people money, delivering better care, and practicing in a unique way. The message resonated with me, but at that time I was pursuing a faculty position at a residency program because I enjoyed teaching so much. Suffice it to say that I filed this "Direct Primary Care" concept in the back of my mind.

Between my second and third years of residency, I went to the Michigan Academy of Family Physicians (MAFP) annual meeting in Traverse City. It was July 2015. There I met Dr. Clint Flanagan of Nextera Healthcare in the Boulder, Colorado area. He spoke passionately about the value of being a primary care doctor and the tremendous value that we provide for our patients. His enthusiasm for the profession came through in a way that I hadn't experienced before.

These two leaders in the field of Direct Primary Care served as a contrast to the typically burnt out and grumbling physician that I had met thus far in training. Even the best doctors grumbled about paperwork, prior authorizations, late patients, packed schedules, and all of the other difficult parts of being a primary care doctor.

It seemed as though we borrowed too much from Henry Ford's assembly line and treated patient visits more like a commodity rather than a genuine human interaction. These transactional relationships in medicine caused me pain – it hurt every time I couldn't give my full time or attention to a patient in need.

At that point, I knew that I would pursue a unique practice model. It only made sense – less-than-fulfilled physicians practicing in a less-than-ideal system surrounded me and I knew that life could be better on the other side.

Additionally, I always had an inner drive to deliver medicine in a more equitable and just system. In short, I wanted to *be the change* that I wanted to see in the healthcare system. Direct Primary Care seemed to align with my values as an individual and as a doctor, but I needed to dive deeper.

So, as an elective rotation, I drove out to Wichita and Denver, and spent a week learning from both Drs. Umbehr and Flanagan. I kicked the tires, took copious notes, and tried to bring the best of their practices to my community in Detroit, Wayne County, and Southeast Michigan.

Now it's August 2018 - about five years after I had initially heard of "Direct Primary Care." I'm living DPC every day, taking care of people of all ages and stages in my clinic in Southwest Detroit. Our youngest patient is about seven months old, and our oldest has 91 years of experience. I answer text messages whenever I receive them, take care of urgent concerns, coordinate care with specialists, and provide primary care services for small businesses.

I am able to do this - to be the doctor that I was

meant to be - because I am a Direct Primary Care doctor. This book is about Direct Primary Care, how we define Direct Primary Care and what is offered in a typical DPC practice. But it's also about inspiration, what inspired me, and what continues to inspire me.

I am inspired by the fact that I can help people with real healthcare needs either in my office or over the phone, or via video chat or email. I am inspired by the fact that I am able to serve people who haven't seen a doctor in years, because we've lowered the cost barriers and therefore have made our service more accessible. I'm inspired by the fact that we can do so much good in such a small space.

I am also inspired by the potential for Plum Health DPC to grow, and to serve more people in our immediate community and across the region. I'm inspired by the happy patients that I get to work with everyday.

I've had great mentors along the way, specifically from the pioneers in the Direct Primary Care world, and I'm grateful for their help in getting me to a successful and sustainable DPC practice.

I wrote this book in order to explain the ethos of Direct Primary Care in greater detail to those interested in knowing more. Those who will benefit from reading this book include individuals who want this type of health care for their families, small business owners who want DPC for their employees, primary care doctors who are thinking of starting their own DPC practices, and all other community stakeholders who are interested in lowering the cost and improving the quality of health care in America.

A sincere thank you for reading,

Paul Thomas, MD
Physician with Plum Health DPC
PlumHealthDPC.com

CHAPTER 1

THE CURRENT CRISIS IN PRIMARY CARE

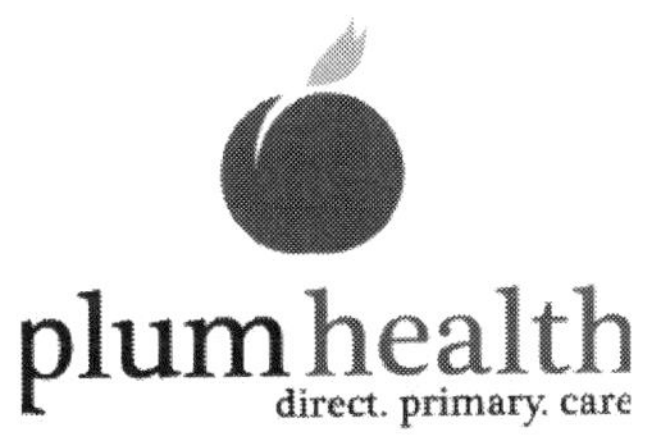

CHAPTER ONE

THE CURRENT CRISIS IN PRIMARY CARE

In high school, I started volunteering at a free clinic in the Cass Corridor. I was working with medical students from Wayne State and taking care of the most vulnerable population in Detroit.

We were supervised by a family doctor and I was always impressed with his ability to solve even the most challenging cases. I wanted to have that kind of skill when I grew up. This is when I decided that I wanted to be a doctor.

In medical school, I became acutely aware of the lack of primary care resources in the city of Detroit. There are only 100 primary care doctors for all 630,000 Detroit residents. That means there's roughly one doctor for every 6,300 people. Essentially all of Detroit is medically underserved.

I wanted to make a difference, to be a part of the solution, but I didn't know what that solution would look like. There wasn't a clear path to being the doctor that I wanted to be, and I was continually frustrated with the broken healthcare system as I progressed from pre-medical student, to medical student, to resident physician.

The further and further I progressed in my training, the less and less time I was able to spend with my patients. Being a primary care doctor in the current healthcare system is like trying to catch sand, with each grain representing a patient concern – there are only so many concerns that we can address before problems start slipping through our fingers.

Prescriptions go unfilled, screening tests are missed, and in many cases the basic healthcare needs of our patients go unmet. Additionally, doctors are feeling burnt out and wanting to leave the profession. I was burnt out, and I hadn't even finished residency.

I was worried that I'd be trapped in a system that undervalues primary care, a system that undervalues human relationships. I was worried that I'd be trapped in a profession that was slowly losing its soul.

The Primary Care Crisis

Primary care in the United States is in crisis. Patients have long wait times, there are too few doctors, and doctors are feeling burned out. These issues are important to address because they give a framework for the current state of health care in America.

Long Wait Times to See Your Primary Care Physician

According to a study by Merritt Hawkins, it takes an average of 24 days to get an appointment with your primary care physician. This wait time varies regionally. Boston has the longest wait time, where it takes an average of 109 days to see a family physician.

There is speculation as to what has caused this. Some suggest more folks with health insurance and an aging population as principal contributors. Whatever the cause, these long wait times can be extremely frustrating for patients.

Unfortunately, current projections indicate that by 2030, the US will be short by 104,900 physicians.

Physician Burnout

Many of my colleagues in primary care now feel as I did during my training – burned out. In fact, a 2016 study performed by Medscape found 51% of physicians experience burnout. Burnout is defined as a loss of enthusiasm for work, feelings of cynicism, and a low sense of personal accomplishment.

There are several complex factors that are pushing doctors towards burnout. They include longer work days, high student debt loads, less time with patients, burdensome electronic medical record (EMR) documentation requirements, pressure for perfection, and perhaps a loss of autonomy.

Not only is burnout affecting doctors, but it is also affecting their patients. From Medical Economics, "research solidly correlates physician burnout with disruptive behavior, increased medical errors, lower patient satisfaction scores, and increased malpractice risk."

High Patient Volumes

The average family physician has roughly 2,400 patients

in their care. This works out to roughly 24 patient visits each day. If this seems like too much for one person to manage, it is. Regrettably, this patient overload is borne out by poor patient outcomes. Findings from a study in the Annals of Family Medicine reveals that patients only receive 55% of recommended chronic and preventive services. Primary care docs struggle to manage high blood pressure, cholesterol levels, blood sugar levels, and other chronic conditions effectively.

This is not the fault of the individual doctor. I repeat: *this is not the fault of the individual doctor.* These are excellent physicians practicing in an unsustainable model of care. Put simply, great docs in a bad system.

In fact, I believe that we should move away from the term "physician burnout" as it places too much blame on the individual doctor, like a light bulb that has gone bad. Rather, physician burnout happens because of systems-based practice problems, and by using terminology reflective of these system failings we will accelerate our ability to identify and solve these challenges.

The aforementioned study goes on to recommend one of two options: either reduce the number of patients to a final number of 200 – 600 per doctor, or keep the patient load the same and lean heavily on ancillary support systems. That second option would look like having a short visit with a doctor, then a consultation with a nutritionist, then a discussion with a therapist, then a visit with the pharmacist to fill medications, followed by a blood draw with the phlebotomist.

In this book, I argue that one of these models is superior to the other. But I will leave you in suspense for the moment. There are other shortcomings in the current healthcare system that we need to discuss first.

An Unfriendly System for Consumers

Health care is one of the few industries that has not undergone seismic changes with the advent of technology. Traditional businesses like the hotel industry and the taxi industry have been upended by technology-enabled disruptors in the free marketplace, like Airbnb and Uber.

Issues like high and unclear pricing, long wait times, limited access to physicians, inconvenient locations, and limited hours have frustrated healthcare consumers. However, there hasn't been a single disrupting force in the marketplace to solve these issues for the majority of consumers or to deliver a better healthcare product.

Urgent care clinics address some of these issues – they typically have a limited wait time and longer hours, some offer clear pricing for cash-pay services, and they tend to have convenient locations. However, urgent care services are lower value because they are not coordinated with longer-term primary care services and thus tend to be disjointed.

Telehealth applications also give consumers shorter wait times and more on-demand services. However, the value here is limited because physicians are unable to perform a physical exam and diagnostic services. Also, these services are not coordinated with primary care services - the medical records from the telehealth visit are not routinely shared with the medical record system of your primary care doc.

Concierge medicine offers on-demand primary care services for patients, but it typically comes at a very high price tag. According to the New York Times, the average annual cost for concierge medicine is $4,000 - $8,000 per year[1]. While concierge medicine offers a high level

1 http://bit.ly/ConciergeMedicineNYT

of service, it is cost-prohibitive for the vast majority of American families.

In short, the healthcare ecosystem is ripe for disruption. If a product or a service could create a better customer experience, more flexible hours and points of contact, and maintain continuity of care, major disruption could occur. This could improve care, save costs, and bring us one step closer to a better healthcare system.

You Can't Text Your Doctor

In the traditional model of care, or the fee-for-service system, doctors are only paid if they have a face-to-face visit with their patients. This means that they will not be paid by the insurance company if they call, text, or email you.

According to the Pew Research Center[2], 82% of Americans own cell phones. And as of May 2010, 72% of American adults send and receive text messages.

Now contrast that to the number of physicians who text their patients. In a 2014 survey[3], only 15% of

2 http://bit.ly/CellPhone-PewResearch
3 http://bit.ly/AAFP-Telehealth

1,557 family physician respondents said that they used telehealth services as an adjunct to face-to-face care.

This is a huge missed opportunity! Texting is fast, direct, and simple. Texting has already been proven to improve health behaviors[4], like smoking cessation, sunscreen use, medication adherence, and increased activity levels. However, it has not been broadly adopted in the traditional or fee-for-service healthcare system.

Inefficiencies in the Fee-For-Service System

If your primary care physician has to see 24 patients each day, they will have to see a new patient every 20 minutes during an 8 hour working day. Therefore, they will have about 20 minutes to focus on you and your needs.

Unfortunately, there are onerous documentation platforms that doctors have to use, called electronic medical records or EMRs. Consequently, that 20-minute appointment is typically fragmented into 8-10 minutes of face time with the doctor and 10-12 minutes of the doctor "charting" or entering all of the requisite information into the EMR behind the scenes.

---

4 http://bit.ly/UoMTextingStudy

One study showed that doctors are spending more than half of their time on administrative tasks[5], or less than half of their time actually taking care of patients.

Further, there are logistical challenges to running a primary care office. A typical primary care office visit costs $150. The doctor will have to send that charge to the insurance company, requiring additional staff to complete this transaction. In addition to the typical medical assistants, nurses, receptionists, and office manager that a doctor employs, they now must also have a dedicated staff of billers and coders to ensure charges are collected.

Even worse, the insurance company or government entity (Medicare or Medicaid) may pay only 60% of what is billed. So for that $150 office visit charge, the doctor may only bring in $90 in revenue. And, in order to pay for all of the support staff to collect on this charge, there is a high overhead to running a fee-for-service primary care office. Typical overhead for a fee-for-service office is 50%.

You might be thinking: "big deal, doctors make enough money anyways – who cares if they have a high

5 http://bit.ly/Forbes-Dr-Time

overhead or if the government doesn't pay them their due?" Because of these inefficiencies in the primary care system, doctors see more and more patients to make up for the lost revenue.

This directly affects you, your family, and the healthcare services that you receive, because you are now shoehorned into a 10-minute appointment. Your health concerns go unaddressed, medications go unfilled, screening tests are forgotten – there simply isn't enough time to be comprehensive.

During my TEDxDetroit talk in November 2017[6], I talked about this exact issue. My grandfather had overgrown toenails and visited his primary care doc to have them trimmed. Only having 8-12 minutes for the visit, the primary care doc referred my grandfather to the podiatrist. Three weeks after visiting the podiatrist, my grandfather received a bill for $350. You see, his Medicare covers primary care visits, but not specialist visits like the visit with the podiatrist.

If the primary care physician had enough time to address the issue fully, it could have prevented a

6 http://bit.ly/DrPaul-TEDx-Nov17

referral and the additional expense therein. Worse still, my grandfather is a retiree on a fixed income – these unforeseen costs can be damaging. Finally, my grandpa is stubborn, and the next time he has an issue, he may hesitate to discuss the problem.

Why Primary Care is Important

Excellent primary care is crucial to the health of individuals, families, communities, and our nation. Importantly "primary care doctor" is an umbrella term that encompasses family medicine doctors, internal medicine doctors, pediatricians, and sometimes obstetricians/gynecologists.

Primary care docs are the first line of care. They order screening tests, can diagnose colds and flus, manage hypertension and diabetes, and take care of broken bones and lacerations. They receive seven years or more of training after college, and are well equipped to handle 80-90% of a person's healthcare needs.

Primary care docs are also the quarterbacks of the healthcare team. They order diagnostic tests via labs or through imaging centers, make referrals to specialist physicians, and ensure that treatment among different sub-specialists doesn't overlap or cause harm.

They are also the backbone of our American healthcare system because of the tremendous value that they offer to communities. A well known report from the American College of Physicians (ACP)[7] reveals the following statistics: for every one additional primary care physician per 10,000 people, there are 5.5% fewer hospital admissions, 11% fewer ER visits, and 7% fewer surgeries.

So, Can't We Just Make More Primary Care Doctors?

As you can see, having more primary care physicians would be beneficial for both individuals and communities. So, why not just make more of them?

Well, primary care is relatively undesirable for medical students. Medical students graduate with an average student loan debt of $190,000 and choosing a higher paying specialty like orthopedic surgery, dermatology, or cardiology makes more financial sense.

It matters how we compensate physicians, and primary care doctors like pediatricians and family docs

7 http://bit.ly/ACP-DPC-Data

are the lowest paid among physicians[8].

Also, it takes about 10 years to train a primary care doctor! Required pre-medical course work, medical school, and residency training takes time. Additionally, there are limited residency positions because of a limited federal budget to train would-be primary care doctors.[9]

Add an aging primary care workforce with more doctors retiring and difficulties like physician burnout as previously discussed, and you have a recipe for this current primary care crisis.

---

8 http://bit.ly/Medscape-Dr-Pay2017

9 http://bit.ly/AAMC-Dr-Shortage

CHAPTER TWO

AN OVERVIEW OF DIRECT PRIMARY CARE

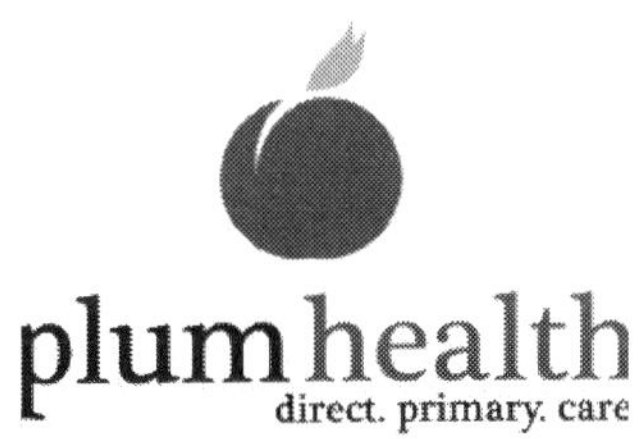

CHAPTER TWO

AN OVERVIEW OF DIRECT PRIMARY CARE

I was worried that I'd be trapped in a system that undervalues primary care, a system that undervalues human relationships. I was worried that I'd be trapped in a profession that was slowly losing its soul.

And that's when I found out about a courageous group of doctors that believe what I believe: that health care should be affordable and accessible for everyone. They call themselves Direct Primary Care doctors because they work directly with their patients.

It's a membership model for health care, where patients can see their doctor whenever they need to. These doctors limit their practice to 500 members, which enables them to provide the best care and avoid burnout.

DPC Docs now have enough time to be with their

patients and to be advocates for their patients. They often get wholesale medications, at cost lab tests, and at-cost imaging studies, which saves their patients thousands of dollars each year.

My story is the story of learning from these doctors, finding the courage to start my own Direct Primary Care practice, and delivering the type of healthcare services that I can be proud of. Our story is about restoring the doctor-patient relationship, and perhaps saving the soul of medicine itself.

Fast Facts

Direct Primary Care connects patients and doctors directly by using a membership model for health care. It sounds really simple because it is. Direct Primary Care succeeds where the fee-for-service system fails. It removes third-party payers, reduces the doctor's patient load, removes barriers between patients and their doctors, and simplifies workflow.

According to recent data from Hint Health[10], there are about 250,000 Americans enrolled in Direct Primary

10 https://www.hint.com/

Care practices and there are roughly 750 DPC practices[11] across the country.

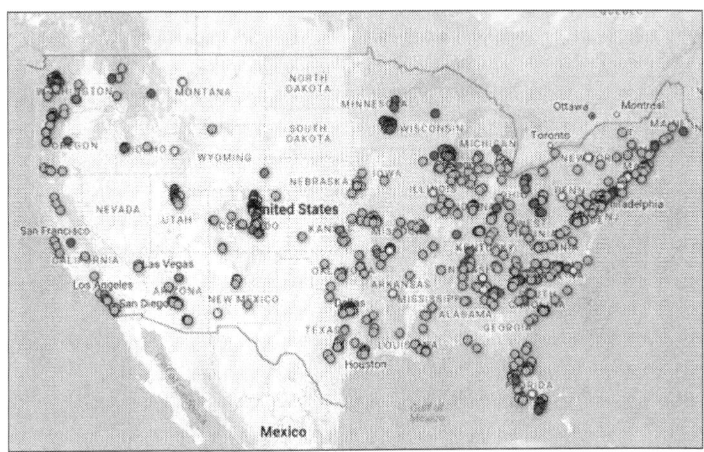

States with the highest per-capita DPC adoption include Colorado, Maine, Kansas, Washington, New Mexico, Idaho, and Texas.

Typical membership prices for Direct Primary Care practices range between $10/month and $100/month. DPC practices usually have tiered pricing based on age. Average adult membership price is $82/month and median adult membership price is $65/month.

According to DPC Frontier[12], a leading resource for

11 http://www.dpcfrontier.com/mapper/

12 http://www.dpcfrontier.com/defined/

DPC doctors, a DPC practice must: charge a periodic fee, not bill any third parties on a fee-for-service basis, and not charge any per visit charge that is greater than the periodic fee.

Let's break this down. DPC doctors charge a periodic fee, and that's the monthly membership cost, like $50 per month. Some docs may choose to charge quarterly or annually. DPC docs do not charge any third party payers for services, meaning that your insurance will not cover the price of the membership.

Direct Primary Care doctors will not bill on a fee-for-service basis. This fee-for-service system is the traditional system where visits last only 20 minutes and the bill is $150 per visit. This is the transactional service that DPC doctors and their patients are attempting to escape.

DPC doctors will not charge a per visit fee that is greater than the periodic fee. Some practices are set up with a monthly membership charge of $50 per month and a per visit fee of $10. In this example, it wouldn't be Direct Primary Care if the per visit fee was $60 and the membership remained $50 per month.

What's Typically Included

As a guiding principle, DPC doctors strive to provide a tremendous amount of value. "Value over volume" as we say. We want to make the membership cost worthwhile for you, your family, and your employees. It starts with being easily accessible, by phone, text, email, and in-person visits.

The majority of DPC doctors do not charge a per visit fee, i.e. all visits are included in the monthly membership price. Some states restrict physicians from dispensing medication, but most doctors offer wholesale medications through their offices. At-cost labs, at-cost imaging services, and some procedures may be included as well.

On a more human level, DPC doctors offer assurance that someone is available for you when you need it most. Sometimes I tell folks that my DPC practice offers assurance, not insurance.

As a caveat, every Direct Primary Care practice is different. Each physician has their own practice philosophy, strengths, weaknesses, and therefore service offerings.

More Time With Your Doctor

One of the most valuable parts of the Direct Primary Care model is more time between patients and their doctors. Typically, people are able to spend an hour with their DPC doctor. This allows more time to develop a trusting relationship that can lead to a more therapeutic interaction. There is inherent value in having a relationship with a primary care physician, and there may be cost savings as well, according to an article in the New York Times Magazine[13].

When patients have more time to talk with their doctors, they reveal more information about their medical history, daily habits, desired outcomes, and other psycho-social issues that may affect their health and wellbeing.

Doctors have more time to listen and more time to ask insightful questions, which allows them to perform at their highest level. They can also use this extra time to counsel patients on improving lifestyle habits, discuss the expected course of a disease process, or inform their patients about the expected effects and side effects of a medication regimen.

13 http://bit.ly/NYT-PC-Value

The essence of Direct Primary Care is this strong relationship between patient and physician. Simply put, Direct Primary Care restores the doctor-patient relationship.

You Can Now Text Your Doctor

Because of the membership model, patients and doctors are no longer confined to that brief office visit. Doctors and patients can now communicate in a way that is unrestricted by insurance company mandates or government regulations.

You can now text your doctor whenever you want. You may send over concerns that you want to address fully at your next scheduled visit, a photo of a rash, or the name of that medication you couldn't remember during your last visit. Your doctor may respond with advice, recommendations, or behavior modification reminders.

This one tool that we all have in our pocket makes medical care far more *accessible*. Patients and doctors may also use email, phone calls, video chat, or other messaging applications to achieve this goal of easy accessibility.

Again, DPC docs strive to deliver a tremendous amount of value, and what's more valuable than a physician that's only a text message away?

Same-Day and Next-Day Appointments

As doctors who practice Direct Primary Care have reduced their patient load, they are now able to leave more time in their day to see urgent appointments. Many DPC docs guarantee same-day or next-day appointments for their members.

This is how urgent issues are supposed to be handled, by your primary care physician. They know you well, your medical history, your allergies, and prior treatments that have succeeded or failed. When DPC docs are reliable and easily accessible, they can eliminate your needs for urgent care or telehealth services.

In contrast, our current system often forces people to use an urgent care or telehealth service in addition to their primary care doctor when an unexpected illness or accident occurs. There are now roughly 9,800 Urgent Care centers in the United States, up 14% since 2008[14].

---

14 http://bit.ly/Urgent-Care-Centers

I would argue that the growth of urgent care is a symptom of a failed primary care system. If patients had easy access to their trusted primary care physician in their hour of greatest need, these ancillary services would cease to be useful.

DPC doctors amend this flaw in the healthcare ecosystem. They are knowledgeable about you and your medical history, caring for you on a long-term basis, as well as available for you should an urgent issue arise.

The Ethics of Providing Affordable Health Care

One of the principal precepts of bioethics is "primum non nocere," or "first, do no harm." As physicians, we took the Hippocratic Oath, stating aloud "I will abstain from all intentional wrong-doing and harm."

As a physician working in a low-income community, my mission is to deliver affordable healthcare services. I will abstain from all intentional wrong-doing and *financial* harm.

Therefore, I will go to great lengths to ensure that the health care that I deliver is not only evidence-based and timely, but also affordable for the people that I serve. Many of my colleagues in the DPC community share this ethos.

Price Transparency

As a part of that "value over volume" mantra, DPC doctors advocate on behalf of their patients and work tirelessly to secure lower prices for the medications and tests that their patients require. They in turn make these prices transparent for their communities.

Many DPC doctors set up contracts with medication wholesalers. These are the same wholesalers who provide medications for big box retail pharmacies. However, DPC doctors do not inflate the price of medications dispensed from their offices and therefore don't make money by providing these medications.

In contrast, the retail pharmacy's main source of income is this profit margin between the wholesale price and the retail price, which inflates the cost of your health care.

Therefore, your DPC doctor can now order the medication that you need and provide the convenience of stocking that medication in their office. This can save you a trip, the price inflation, and the wait time associated with going to the retail pharmacy.

Similarly DPC docs contract with national laboratories and imaging centers to provide at-cost testing. When patients pay cash for these services, savings can range from 50-90%. Most importantly, these prices become transparent and patients can make more informed decisions about their healthcare expenditures. Read on for concrete examples in Chapter Three.

Removing Inefficiencies

Direct Primary Care practices remove inefficiencies from the healthcare system. DPC docs leverage texting and emails to make communication more streamlined.

Further, DPC docs bill their patients directly, removing health insurance companies from the primary care equation. Billing your insurance company takes several man-hours, which can inflate the cost of health care by 10-20%.

DPC doctors also remove inefficient electronic medical record (EMR) systems from their practices. As an anecdote, one doctor in the fee-for-service system used 32 clicks to order one flu shot![15] In contrast, the documentation in DPC clinics is streamlined. The medical note is truly a note for the doctor and the patient, and not a series of check boxes and form data to optimize billing and coding for insurance reimbursement.

By removing these inefficiencies, DPC doctors are now able to focus on what is truly important: the doctor-patient relationship.

Happy Patients + Happy Doctors = Direct Primary Care

Now that you've learned more about Direct Primary Care, you can see how different people benefit in different ways in this model. This section is a hat tip to Dr. Clint Flanagan, who inspired me when he gave a lecture at the Michigan Academy of Family Physicians annual conference in July 2015.

Dr. Flanagan made the journey all the way from his home and his practice in the Boulder, Colorado area to teach other doctors in Michigan about Direct Primary Care. The title of this section was the title of his

15 http://bit.ly/EHR-Burdens

presentation: "Happy Patients + Happy Doctors = Direct Primary Care."

And now, you can see why this is the case! Patients are happy because they have more time with their doctor. Having enough time to address all of my patients' concerns in one sitting is tremendously valuable for my members, especially when they have chronic conditions or complex medical problems. Having this time is also valuable for me, because I can engage in more complex thinking and decision-making, rather than having a disjointed experience over multiple visits.

Patients are able to call, text and email their doctor at any time. For me, I always have my cell phone in my pocket and I am reachable at virtually any hour. For my patients, they have the knowledge and assurance that I will be responsive to them when something arises.

Patients also get the best prices on medications, laboratory services, and imaging services. We buy wholesale medications and dispense them out of our office, saving our members thousands of dollars each month. We also draw blood in our office and negotiate frequently with our lab services company for the best prices. Also, we work with an imaging service company for the best prices on diagnostic imaging, from mammograms to x-rays and CT scans.

As a result of the increased satisfaction that comes from practicing in this model, I have experienced much less burnout than during my training in the fee-for-service system. This translates to better interactions with my patients and increased satisfaction for the patients that I serve.

CHAPTER THREE

DETAILS ABOUT PLUM HEALTH DPC

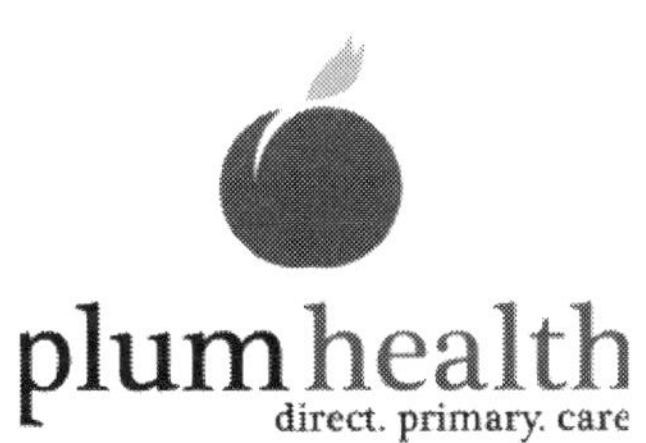

CHAPTER THREE

DETAILS ABOUT PLUM HEALTH DPC

My story is the story of learning from these Direct Primary Care doctors, finding the courage to start my own DPC practice, and delivering the type of healthcare services that I can be proud of. Our story is about restoring the doctor-patient relationship, and perhaps saving the soul of medicine itself.

Now that I have been practicing in a Direct Primary Care model, I want to share what I've learned. I want to share my story with the broader community and help others understand Direct Primary Care and what it entails.

The illustrative examples in this chapter are given in order to move the discussion from theoretical to practical. The stories are shared with permission from my patients, although the details are changed to protect their identities.

Wholesale Medications at Plum Health DPC

At Plum Health DPC, we offer wholesale medications for our patients who are members of the practice. We have a broad selection of medications that grows as we add more members. When a new member signs up for our service, we evaluate their current medications, decide which type of therapy is best to continue, and order whichever medication is needed.

Additionally, we save our members roughly 50 – 90% on the cost of their medications. We typically purchase medications in bulk, purchasing 1000 pills at a time. For example Amlodipine 5 mg is 1¢ per pill, Cyclobenzaprine (Flexeril) is 19¢ per pill, Escitalopram (Lexapro) 10 mg is 6¢ per pill, Fluconazole (Diflucan) 150 mg is $1.55 per pill, Furosemide (Lasix) 20 mg is 2¢ per pill, Hydrochlorothiazide (HCTZ) 12.5 mg is 3¢ per pill, Metformin 500 mg is 1.3¢ per pill, Simvastatin (Zocor) 20 mg is 1.9¢ per pill, etc…

Some patients sign up for the service because they are able to save the entire cost of membership based on medication savings alone. I've had a few patients email me the list of their current medications, and I respond with our Plum Health inventory prices as a free consultation.

One of our members came to our clinic because of genital herpes outbreak. This is obviously a sensitive issue – there is still a great deal of stigma and other negative feelings wrapped around a diagnosis like herpes. The patient had gone to the pharmacy and asked for Valacyclovir or Valtrex to combat her ongoing symptoms.

At the pharmacy, she was told that the cost of a course of therapy – six pills – would be $100. She was uninsured, relatively low income and could not afford this price. She heard about our clinic from a local TV news story, and made an appointment to inquire about the medication. At our clinic, Valacyclovir (Valtrex) 500 mg tablets cost 23¢ per pill, so the course of therapy for one outbreak costs $1.38.

At-Cost Labs

Another way that we provide tremendous value for our members at Plum Health DPC is by negotiating for lower prices on lab work.

Currently, our price for a comprehensive list of lab tests is $31. This includes a comprehensive metabolic panel (CMP) for $6, which reveals the kidney function, liver function, blood sugar, and electrolyte levels. It also includes a Hemoglobin A1c level for $6, which reveals the average blood sugar levels over the last 3 months. This panel also measures the Thyroid Stimulating Hormone (TSH) for $6, the Complete Blood Count (CBC) for $4, and the Lipid Panel for $6. The Lipid Panel checks the Total Cholesterol, HDL, LDL, and Triglyceride levels.

For those of you keeping score at home, the above set of labs adds up to $28, but we add on a $3 draw fee so that we can replenish our blood draw supplies.

In contrast, if you were to have this same set of labs drawn through the large hospital system in the region,[16] it would cost roughly $500 billed to your insurance. Now, if you have 80/20 coverage on your insurance plan, the amount of money that you would be responsible for after insurance would be $100. Remember, the actual cost is $28.

---

16 http://bit.ly/PlumHealth-Savings

Or, if you were uninsured and were subject to the same prices as the insurance company, the cost would be $500. This is where price inflation in the medical field is the most harmful, and this is one of the biggest problems in our current healthcare system: fee-for-service billing disproportionately affects those who are uninsured.

We also have the capacity to request any lab test that we need for our patients. We started with a relatively short list of options for lab work, but as we've seen a more diverse group of patients, we have requested and received at-cost prices for several different lab tests.

A Vitamin D level is $16.90, a B12 level is $10, a Folate level is $20, HIV test is $10, Syphilis test is $4, Chlamydia and Gonorrhea testing is $23, blood pregnancy test is $25, a Lyme titer is $45, T3 costs $7, T4 costs $5, Thyroid Peroxidase AB is $10, Testosterone level is $30, etc…

If every healthcare delivery system in America listed their prices, we could provide patients with a broader scope of choices. By listing prices publicly, we are one step closer to creating a free market healthcare ecosystem, which may improve both quality and service in the healthcare industry. With choice comes freedom.

At-Cost Imaging Services

At Plum Health DPC, we also provide at-cost imaging services. We currently contract with a third party imaging services company. During our office visits, if imaging is deemed necessary, an order is written for the imaging service. Our patients then go to the imaging center and pay cash or credit or check at the time of service.

Chest x-rays are $32, ultrasounds are in the $100 - $150 range depending on the body part, MRI tests range from $300 - $600 depending on the body part and the use of contrast, and CT scans are in the range of $200 - $500 again depending on the body part and use of contrast.

This price includes readings from the radiologist on-site, a faxed report and a digital rendering of the imaging test. Typically, the radiology team processes images in 24 hours or less.

As the ordering physician, I have access to an online portal through which I can evaluate the images and discuss the findings with my members. I often take screenshots and include the area of pathology as an attachment in the email to my patients.

Further, I often call the radiologist and have a conversation about the imaging study and how it relates to the person that I am caring for. This can lead to greater insight from both my perspective and the radiologist's perspective, which can lead to a more accurate diagnosis and a more comprehensive treatment plan.

Imaging in Action

This summer, one of my members fell and injured their arm at a music festival – they slipped while dancing. The music festival's on-site doctor diagnosed a shoulder dislocation, but unfortunately missed a small fracture in the humerus or upper arm bone. During the process of realigning the shoulder, the fracture to the humerus worsened.

When the patient came to our office in Detroit, he had notable swelling, bruising, immobility, and pain. He relayed the story about the music festival and the onsite doctor and the dislocation, but something was amiss. You typically don't see that much bruising, immobility, and pain from a re-aligned dislocation. I immediately ordered an MRI of the shoulder and he was able to obtain the imaging service in a few days.

I received the images about 24 hours after they were taken. There were several small injuries that needed to be discussed, but it would be difficult to relay them over the phone. We set up a time to talk later that week when our schedules aligned.

That evening I went to a neighborhood eatery and serendipitously saw my patient, seated at the other end of the restaurant. He waved, and I waved back. I walked over, shook his hand and he invited me to join him at his table. We talked for a few moments and decided that it would be a good time to review the MRI.

We reviewed the information on my smart phone and discussed the different injuries in the shoulder. We also talked about next steps in therapy and a good orthopedic surgeon nearby who would give a sound second opinion.

In-Office Procedures

Family Medicine doctors are trained to perform a broad range of in-office procedures. At Plum Health DPC, we often perform Pap tests, joint injections, shave biopsies, laceration repair, incision and drainage, etc…

We do not bill or charge extra for the time it takes to perform the in-office procedures. However, there may be an additional charge for medications or for pathology fees. For example, we do not charge to perform the Pap test in the office, but in order to have the Pap test read by the pathologist it costs $33.

Even though the suture material and sterile equipment costs roughly $15, laceration repair is on the house, i.e. it's free to sew up your cuts. One of our members put a drill through his palm while working on his house late one Friday evening. I drove in, met him at the office at 9:30 pm, and put 5 stitches into his skin. He left around 9:50 pm without an additional charge. It was during the basketball playoffs and he was excited that he'd actually be able to catch the end of the game.

As for joint injections, these procedures can be billed to insurance companies for roughly $200. However, in our clinic, we only charge for the cost of the medication. We often use Kenalog, which costs roughly $7.50 per mL. So, when we perform a joint injection in the office, the final cost is $7.50.

I remove earwax, freeze warts, and trim toenails for free. We can also perform point-of-care testing like urine pregnancy tests and rapid testing for Strep throat, Influenza A and B, and Mononucleosis.

Pathology Services

Pathology services are available through Plum Health as well. As described above, we ship out Pap tests to a pathologist for a total of $33. Many of our patients have long-standing moles that they would like to have biopsied so that they can attain peace of mind.

For simple skin biopsies of concerning moles or pedunculated growths, pathology charges are $69. The shipping is typically done overnight, and the readings come back within 1 week from the pathologist.

When to Use Health Insurance

Although cars and people are very different, I find the auto insurance analogy interesting and a reasonable way to explain Direct Primary Care as it relates to health insurance. The idea is this: we all have to have auto insurance, which is a financial tool that we use to protect us from financial loss in the case of an accident or catastrophe.

Yet, for the rest of our cars' needs, we use the marketplace for maintenance and enhancements. If we need gas for our cars, we buy it at a gas station and we typically check the local prices for comparison, by using an app or scanning the prices on our drive home.

When our tires are worn after 30,000 miles, we replace them. Sometimes we shop around for the best "deal", and sometimes we need to replace a tire urgently in the case of a flat. Likewise, if we wanted to enhance our car for optimal performance, we use the marketplace to make an informed purchase. This may range from an oil change to a new transmission or exhaust system.

Importantly, we don't use our car insurance to pay for oil changes or new wiper blades.

The overarching view of health care from the DPC perspective is that free-market principles should apply. Again, health insurance should be a financial tool to protect you from financial ruin in the case of an accident, heart attack, or stroke. The coverage that you should purchase depends on your comfort with risk, i.e. you may feel comfortable paying a higher premium each month for a lower deductible or vice versa.

Likewise, other services in the healthcare marketplace should be available for purchase. Services like flu shots, physical exams, Pap tests, sick visits, etc… should be available to be bought in the free market.

To some extent, this is already happening. Healthcare consumers are able to purchase flu shots at big box pharmacies for $29.99 and most urgent care centers charge a flat visit price of $100 per visit. But, price transparency in the healthcare marketplace are far from robust.

Further, it does not make sense to buy insurance for primary care services. Insurance is meant for big, unforeseen expenses, not routine services. Primary care services are less expensive and delivered at a higher level of quality when paid for directly. Asking a third party payer, like a large insurance company or Medicare, to pay for primary care services only inflates the cost of care and decreases quality and transparency.

Fortunately, Direct Primary Care clinics are making prices for healthcare services more transparent for consumers. DPC clinics, shared savings plans for health care, as well as surgery centers that display their prices like the Surgery Center of Oklahoma are restoring free-market forces in the healthcare ecosystem.

My argument is that these free market principles will improve patient choice, decrease cost, and make physicians and healthcare systems more responsive to patient needs.

Pragmatically, as a member of my service at Plum Health DPC, we can leverage whichever resources are available in the marketplace to get you the best price and the best quality.

As an example, if you need a chest x-ray, it will likely be less expensive and less of a hassle to purchase it at the cash price of $32. However, if major surgery is required, using your health insurance may be the best option. If you have a high premium, low deductible health insurance plan, then using your insurance for the expensive procedure is likely your best option. But, if you have a low premium, high deductible plan, you may save money by paying cash for the expensive procedure.

These can be complex and difficult decisions, but part of my job is to be an advocate for you, your health, and your financial wellness. I will take the time to review the available choices and together we can make a decision about the best option.

Radical Price Transparency

In this Direct Primary Care model, we want to deliver as much value as possible. To that end, we don't make any money on the medications, laboratory, or imaging services that we provide through Plum Health DPC. The only way that we make money is through the memberships.

There are no upcharges, there are no middlemen, and you have the satisfaction of knowing exactly where your healthcare dollars are going. As I've mentioned before, I believe that price transparency in the healthcare ecosystem will improve the choice and therefore the quality of services for individuals, families, and small businesses in our country.

Leveraging Online Platforms for Specialty Consultations

As a board certified Family Medicine doctor, I am able to care for 80 – 90% of what an individual may need in terms of healthcare services. Family Medicine doctors care for a broad spectrum of patients and a broad range of conditions.

That 10-20% outside of my scope of practice includes services like colonoscopies, major surgeries, and delivering babies.

One way that I extend my scope of practice is by leveraging an online consultation platform called RubiconMD. On this platform, there are over 200 medical specialists of whom we can ask questions, from Endocrinologists who specialize in Thyroid dysfunction, to Psychiatrists who specialize in sleep disorders, to Dermatologists who specialize in skin lesions and many more.

So, if there's a case that's outside of my comfort zone, I can write up a consult to the appropriate specialist and receive feedback, typically within 24 hours. Of note, this service is free-of-charge to our members at Plum Health.

Leveraging Local Resources for Other Tests and Consults

One of the beautiful aspects of this Direct Primary Care model is that I have time to advocate for my patients. For example, if one of my patients needs a medical service that I cannot provide, I can call around to my local physician colleagues and ask for at-cost pricing.

I suspected heart failure in one of my members, but had no way of performing an echocardiogram, or an ultrasound of the heart to measure its contractions and relaxations. I needed this test to make an accurate diagnosis. So, I called a local, independent cardiologist and he was able to perform the test for $137.

I also had a patient who needed a sleep study. I called a local, independent pulmonologist and asked for their cash prices for sleep studies. Their at-home sleep studies cost $250 and their in-office sleep studies are $500. This includes interpretation.

This technique doesn't work as well with large hospital systems. It is often easier to receive cash prices from independent physicians than from larger hospital organizations with more layers of bureaucracy.

Texting Our Patients to Motivate Change

At Plum Health we like to guide people to better lifestyle choices. For example, if you're trying to quit smoking, we can help you by reminding you of your commitment.

How do we do this? It's really simple, actually. We just send you a text message! There is a great deal of evidence to support these types of interventions. There is a meta analysis on Text Messaging-Based Interventions for Smoking Cessation in the Journal of Medical Internet Research that came to this conclusion: "The current meta-analytic review provides unequivocal support for the efficacy of text messaging interventions for smoking abstinence."

Further, texting patients about their health can have different applications. For example, a text message to a patient regarding their exercise patterns or medication adherence can help them to achieve their goals. It's exciting to leverage these simple tools to be compassionately connected with my patients.

On Being Easily Accessible

Even on the weekends and holidays, we try to be as accessible as possible for our patients. For example, we took on a new patient on the last Sunday in November 2017. They had developed a serious abscess in their armpit over that Thanksgiving weekend. On their drive home, they realized that they should probably have it evaluated.

Because it was a Sunday evening, they knew that it would be difficult to find an available doctor in Detroit. They searched "Doctor Open Today" on Google and fortunately found our Plum Health clinic.

The patient called around 2:30 pm on Sunday, and I was able to see them in the office 2 hours later. We drained the abscess and started the appropriate antibiotic, dispensed from our in-clinic pharmacy. They had a follow up appointment during regular business hours on Tuesday, and they were feeling much better.

On Christmas Eve 2017, one of our patients developed a throat issue. She is a professional singer for a church in Detroit, and was expected to sing for the Christmas Eve and Christmas Day services. She sent me a text around 1 pm on Christmas Eve, and I was able to meet her at the office at 1:30 pm.

I performed an examination and got her the medications that she needed to power through her remaining two performances. I am sincerely happy to help people in these types of situations, and happy to be a trusted resource for my patients in their time of need.

Helping People Navigate the Complex Medical System

I unequivocally recommend that my patients carry an insurance plan, and I encourage folks to have the type of insurance plan that they are comfortable with. For those members who have few chronic medical conditions and a low rate of hospital utilization, a low-premium, high-deductible plan is recommended.

This way, they have the potential to save a significant amount of money each year by pairing a lower-cost insurance policy with the Direct Primary Care services at Plum Health DPC.

As my members become more comfortable with my practice, they realize that they can tailor their level of insurance coverage to compliment the primary care services that they receive through Plum Health.

Helping Businesses Navigate Complex Coverage Decisions

As more individuals have signed up, the word has spread about the type of work that we do at Plum Health DPC. Our first members have become advocates for our service. Once they experience what it's like to be a patient with Plum Health, they tend to want to tell their family, friends, neighbors, and coworkers.

Recently we've had the privilege of taking care of employer groups. We are able to give a discounted rate to larger groups of employees, providing tremendous value for both the employer and the employees. Often times, these employer groups are small businesses that aren't able to afford traditional health insurance for their staff, but want to offer some kind of healthcare service.

All of the services that individuals receive through Plum Health DPC are also given to the employees who sign up through one of these employer group contracts. Typically, the employer will invite us to meet with all of their employees. We'll go over the program and if it's a good fit, we will go forward with enrolling the employer group.

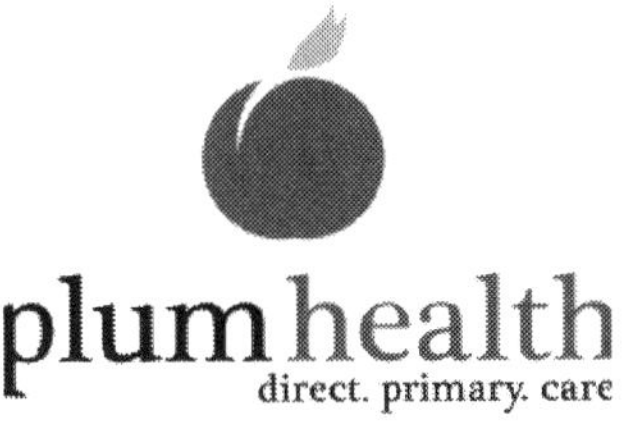

So, Why Plum?

Now that you understand more about the services that we offer at Plum Health, you may be interested to know why we chose a Plum as our logo. For us, a Plum is healthy. It fits in your hand. It's purple. It's simple. It's two overlapping circles.

First, a Plum can be drawn with two overlapping circles. To us, this symbolizes the doctor - patient relationship. At Plum Health, there is more overlap in the relationship between doctor and patient. We believe that having a closer relationship with your doctor can allow you to live a healthier and happier life.

Next, a Plum is a healthy food, and at Plum Health DPC we know that taking better care of yourself begins with what we eat and how we move. The choice of a Plum is inspired by bike rides to Eastern Market, and finding those healthy foods. At Plum Health, we can direct you to healthy resources throughout Detroit and Metro Detroit.

Third, a Plum is simple, it fits in your hand, and you can take it with you. At Plum Health DPC, we have set out to simplify health care for our members. We aim to eliminate the frustrations in the fee-for-service system like waiting too long to see your doctor, confusing billing, and co-pays.

You can also take our services with you. Say you're traveling and something comes up, we can help to guide you through whatever problems you face. Maybe it's talking you through a head cold, reviewing a management plan, or sending a medication that you forgot at home to the pharmacy nearest you.

Finally, a Plum is purple. At Plum Health DPC, we proudly serve and welcome people of all backgrounds. All ages, stages, races, ethnicities, and orientations are welcome. Additionally, our price points for individuals are less than a typical cell phone bill[17] and our price points for families are less than a typical cable bill. This allows us to serve people of all income levels.

---

17 https://www.plumhealthdpc.com/pricing

Fighting for a Greater Good

I also started Plum Health DPC to fight for a greater good. This speaks to our mission, vision, and values. I've mentioned my desire to create a more just and equitable healthcare system, and there are a few ways that I'm addressing this issue.

First, by being a primary care doctor in Detroit, by choosing to locate my practice in Detroit, Michigan, we are already having an impact. As stated previously, there are only 100 primary care physicians in the entire City of Detroit for 633,000 residents. Again, that's 1 primary care doctor for every 6,300 residents! This is horribly underserved, and I want to address this issue head on.

Next, I want to teach and inspire the next generation of doctors to choose primary care and to work in underserved areas. Primary care physicians provide so much value to their communities, and I want to see as many medical students choose Family Medicine as possible.

To this end, I've been a frequent speaker at conferences and medical schools. In July 2017, I was invited to deliver the Keynote Speech[18] at the Wayne State University School of Medicine White Coat Ceremony. This was a tremendous honor!

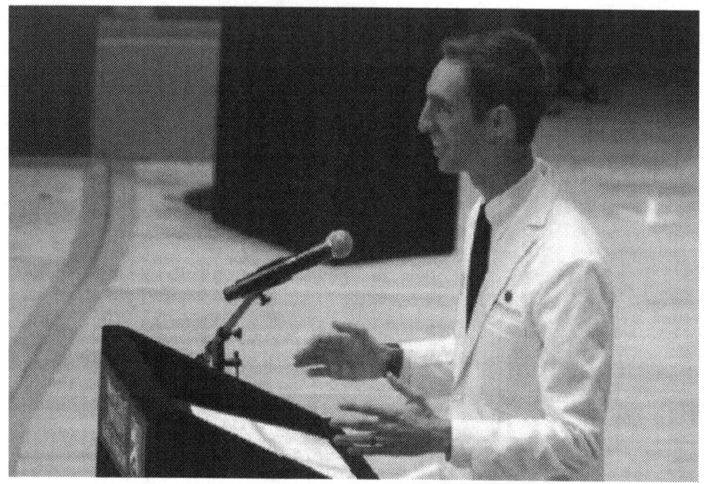

Additionally, I advocate for more primary care resources at the Federal level. In June of 2017, I was able to go to Washington D.C.[19] and speak with a number of Senators and Congressional Representatives about the importance of primary care and about this new model of healthcare delivery.

Finally, I want to educate the community about Direct Primary Care and about Family Medicine. I believe that family medicine doctors and Direct Primary Care doctors are making our world a better place. That's why I

18 http://bit.ly/PlumHealth-073117

19 http://bit.ly/PlumHealth-061517

get out and speak at different events, like TEDxDetroit or write blog posts or op-eds or even this book.

Talking about Direct Primary Care at TEDxDetroit

TEDxDetroit was held on a Thursday evening, November 9th, at the Charles H. Wright Museum for African American History and it was an amazing event. For those of you who don't know, TED stands for Technology, Entertainment, and Design.

From their website, TED is a nonpartisan nonprofit devoted to spreading ideas, usually in the form of short, powerful talks. TED began in 1984 as a conference where Technology, Entertainment and Design converged, and today covers almost all topics — from science to business to global issues — in more than 110 languages. Meanwhile, independently run TEDx events help share ideas in communities around the world.

TEDxDetroit is one of those independently-organized events that brought together thought leaders in Detroit and Southeast Michigan. The topic: ideas worth spreading.

It was an honor to be selected and an honor to share the stage with innovators like Kimberly Dowdell of Century Partners, Jon Rimanelli of AirSpaceX, and Marlin Williams of SistersCode.

To watch the full video, check out our blog at PlumHealthDPC.com/blog.[20]

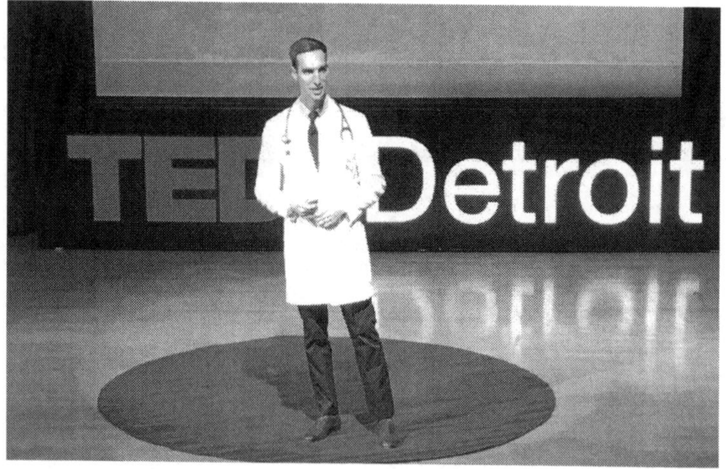

Action Steps

If you are an individual, seeking this type of care, there is an interactive listing of Direct Primary Care doctors at DOCFrontier.com/mapper.[21]

If you are a physician seeking to start this type of practice, participate in the next Direct Primary Care

20 PlumHealthDPC.com/blog.

21 DOCFrontier.com/mapper

conference through the AAFP or the Docs 4 Patient Care Foundation.[22] You can also visit a nearby DPC clinic by using the above mapper tool, or send me an email, paul@plumhealthdpc.com. I'm sincerely happy to guide you on your next step in this journey.

Closing Thoughts

Direct Primary Care, while imperfect, has several advantages over the existing fee-for-service system. The DPC model restores the doctor-patient relationship; it puts the patient at the center of the practice of medicine.

Direct Primary Care empowers doctors to deliver the type of medical care that they can be proud of. We can be proud to serve our family, friends, neighbors and broader community through this model.

Further, broad implementation of DPC may allow individuals, families, businesses, and governments to save roughly 20% on their overall healthcare expenditures.

I look forward, not only to growing Plum Health DPC, but also to the growing Direct Primary Care movement in the United States. As the movement grows,

22 https://d4pcfoundation.org/dpc2017/

we will be that much closer to affordable, accessible healthcare services for everyone.

ACKNOWLEDGMENTS

There is an innumerable list of people that I need to thank for helping me along the way. Two years ago when I first wrote my business plan for Plum Health, I could not imagine how many people I would meet and how many doors that this endeavor would open for me. Here's my thanks to all of those who helped get to this point by lending their skills, wisdom, and expertise.

To Dr. Karen Weaver, for allowing me the freedom to write my business plan in a residency-related practice management course. To all of my co-residents who helped me fortify that plan. To Max Schmidt, who told me to listen to a podcast on free-market healthcare solutions. To Dr. Josh Umbehr, for taking my call, encouraging me to take the leap, and accommodating my visit to ATLAS MD. To Dr. Clint Flanagan for speaking in Michigan at the MAFP annual conference, inspiring me, and hosting me at Nextera Healthcare in Colorado.

To Tommy Daguanno for helping me nail my

branding and website design – your early intervention put me on a solid track for success. To Michelle Graham for the wonderful cover design.

To Mayor Mike Duggan and his administration, especially those involved in the Motor City Match program. To April Boyle of the Build Institute, whose Co-Starters course taught me about starting a business in Detroit. To Nicole Mangis, a great teacher, and all of my classmates at Build. To Faris Alami and the entire staff at TechTown, Ned, Regina, Sarah, Amy, and Bridget, as well as Niles Heron, consultant extrordainare, and my classmates in the Retail Boot Camp course.

To Ingrid Jacques of the Detroit News, for lending a platform to express my opinions on health care. To Mark S. Lee, for interviewing me on Small Talk on CBS Radio as well as in print via his column in Crain's Detroit Business. To Steve Garagiola and his team at Channel 4 News (WDIV Detroit) for the best television news story I've ever seen on Direct Primary Care. To John Bruske, Jackie Berg, Paul Natinsky, Jennifer Hamra, Pamela Hillard Owens, Khary Frazier, and all of the other writers, bloggers, podcasters and journalists who've shared the story of Plum Health DPC.

To the broader DPC community and DPC doctors who are leading the charge to create a better healthcare system for their patients, their communities, and the entire nation.

To the PA Students, Medical Students and Residents who have rotated through the Plum Health clinic, thank you for lending your expertise and thank you for helping me deliver affordable, accessible health care in Detroit.

To all of my patients, the current and former members of Plum Health – thank you for entrusting me with your care. I am continually humbled to have the honor of caring for so many wonderful people.

To Zanuel Moore for the cover photography. To Norman Fletcher for helping take the book from a final draft to the published document that you're reading now.

A huge thank you to all of my alpha readers who gave me tremendous insight and feedback on early drafts of this book. Big ups to Kirk Bennett for informing me of the difference between "healthcare," an adjective, and "health care," a noun. Finally, an apology to all of my high school English teachers – my grammar, punctuation, and tense agreement isn't the best.

Made in the USA
Lexington, KY
27 November 2018